THE LITTL
QUITTING
SMOKING

ALLEN CARR

SIRIUS

SIRIUS

This edition published in 2019 by Sirius Publishing, a division of
Arcturus Publishing Limited,
26/27 Bickels Yard, 151–153 Bermondsey Street,
London SE1 3HA

ISBN: 978-1-78950-099-8
AD000037US

Printed in China

FOREWORD BY JOHN DICEY, GLOBAL CEO AND SENIOR THERAPIST, ALLEN CARR'S EASYWAY

Tasked by Allen with ensuring that his legacy achieves its full potential, we've taken Allen Carr's Easyway from videos to DVD, from clinics to apps, from computer games to audio books, to online programs, video-on-demand, and beyond.

Behind this phenomenal success lies one simple truth—a truth that Allen discovered by chance and passed on to millions of people. What connects us all is that none of us expected to be changed in the way we were. We were all skeptical, all laboring under the same illusions. There's a vast army of smokers and vapers out there still suffering their own private nightmare, believing that they enjoy smoking or vaping, that it provides them with some kind of benefit, and that, as a result, it's hard to quit. It isn't; it's easy.

The truth about smoking is kept hidden from most smokers and even from many ex-smokers. That's why some who quit using willpower continue to crave cigarettes long after they stub out their final cigarette. They believe they are making a sacrifice, resigned to doing without something that provides them with pleasure or support, believing that it helps them to control their weight, to relax, to socialize, and to handle stress. Understanding the simple truth and recognizing how it applies to you is the key to escaping the nicotine trap and staying free permanently. But it takes a special method to do that.

**ALLEN CARR'S EASYWAY
IS THE METHOD THAT WORKS**

INTRODUCTION BY THE AUTHOR

Imagine a drug that causes the premature death of one in two users, costs the average addict $130,000/£100,000 in a lifetime, makes you feel insecure, bored, and tense, tastes foul, ruins your confidence, impedes your concentration, and has no advantages whatsoever.

Can you believe that at one time over 90% of the adult population of western society was addicted to this drug?

Can you imagine yourself becoming addicted to such a drug? If you are a smoker, casual or otherwise, you already are an addict. The drug is nicotine.

Supposing I could convince you that the facts about smoking are exactly as I have described above and, furthermore, that any smoker can find it easy to quit…

IMMEDIATELY AND EASILY

**WITHOUT USING WILLPOWER,
GIMMICKS, OR SUBSTITUTES**

WITHOUT PUTTING ON WEIGHT

If I could further convince you that you won't miss smoking, that you'll enjoy social occasions more, and be better able to cope with stressful situations, would you quit? Then read on. I having nothing but good news for you.

IMPORTANT WARNING!

Unless you have already quit, do not attempt to do so, or even to cut down, before you have read and understood the whole book.

WHEN DID YOU DECIDE
TO BE A SMOKER?

No. I don't mean what was the occasion of your first cigarette, but when did you decide to smoke every day?

Or did you just drift into it like every other smoker on the planet?

WILL YOU ALWAYS BE A SMOKER?

So when will you quit?

> After you've spent the $130,000/£100,000?

> When you've ruined your health?

> When the time is right?

How many years have you smoked?

Do you ever wonder why it never seems the right time
to quit?

WHY DO YOU SMOKE?

Because it tastes good?

> *Do you eat it?*

For something to do with your hands?
> *Try a ballpoint pen.*

For oral satisfaction?
> *Use a pacifier.*

To relieve boredom and stress, and aid relaxation and concentration?

> *Surely boredom and concentration are opposites, and so are stress and relaxation.*

WHICH ARE YOUR FAVORITE CIGARETTES?

First in the morning? *Isn't that the one that tastes the worst?*

After a meal or with a drink, when answering the phone or during moments of stress? *How can an identical cigarette out of the same pack taste different to, or have completely the opposite effect from, the one smoked an hour earlier?*

DO YOU WISH YOUR CHILDREN SMOKED?

If the answer is no, it means that you wish you were a nonsmoker! So why aren't you? *Because smoking is a habit and habits are difficult to break?* Are they?

In the U.S., people are in the habit of driving on the right. But if you drive in Britain, for example, you can break the habit immediately without difficulty.

SO WHY DO SMOKERS CONTINUE TO SMOKE?

For one reason and one reason alone. They have fallen into the most subtle, ingenious trap that man and nature have combined to set:

THEY ARE ADDICTED
TO NICOTINE!

THE MOST POWERFUL DRUG IN THE WORLD!

Nicotine is the most powerful addictive drug known to mankind. Just one cigarette can hook you, particularly if you have been addicted previously.

A POWERFUL POISON!

The nicotine content of just one cigarette injected directly into a vein would kill you. Please don't try it. This is why those first cigarettes make you feel dizzy and sick.

THE NATURE OF THE TRAP

When the nicotine from the first cigarette leaves your body, it creates a feeling of emptiness and insecurity—the feeling that smokers know as "needing a cigarette" or "needing something to do with their hands."

TIGHT SHOES!

If you light another cigarette, the nicotine is replaced, and the empty, insecure feeling immediately disappears. It's the feeling that smokers describe as satisfaction or pleasure.

It's like wearing tight shoes just for the pleasure of taking them off!

THE LIFETIME'S CHAIN

When you extinguish the second cigarette, the nicotine leaves, the empty, insecure feeling returns, and now the smoker needs another and another, ad infinitum, until death do you part!

THE LITTLE MONSTER

Think of that empty feeling as a tape worm inside your body that feeds on nicotine. The true reason that any smoker continues to smoke is to feed that little nicotine monster.

YOU ARE ABOUT TO STARVE IT!

WHY ISN'T ALL THIS OBVIOUS?

Because it works back to front. It's when you aren't smoking that you suffer the craving. The moment you light up it is relieved. Your brain is fooled into believing you receive a genuine pleasure or crutch.

What you are really enjoying is getting back to the state you were in permanently before you lit that first cigarette.

In fact, you are simply trying to feel as relaxed as a nonsmoker!

QUITTING

YOU NEVER GET THERE, UNLESS YOU QUIT!

When you learn to smoke, you are merely teaching your body to become immune to a powerful poison. After a short period you only partially relieve the empty feeling. This is why the tendency is to smoke more and more.

QUITTING

DRUG ADDICTION
OR GENUINE PLEASURE?

Genuine pleasures, like a nice vacation, create no feeling of guilt. We are pleased to boast about them and, while we would like to enjoy the pleasure more often, we do not feel deprived or miserable when not partaking of the pleasure. All smokers brag about how little they smoke, but even the thought of being without cigarettes creates panic.

PICTURE A HEROIN ADDICT

There's a terrible panic when they have no heroin, but a wonderful feeling of "pleasure" when they plunge that hypodermic into a vein. Nonheroin addicts don't suffer that feeling of panic. Heroin doesn't relieve it. **IT CAUSES IT!** Nonsmokers don't suffer the desperate pangs of needing a cigarette. Neither did you before you became addicted to nicotine.

THE INCREDIBLE IRONY OF IT ALL

The only reason you or any other smoker needs or wants a cigarette is to try to get rid of the feeling of nicotine withdrawal. But it is only smokers who suffer from nicotine withdrawal. Nonsmokers do not. So all you are trying to do whenever you light a cigarette is feel like a nonsmoker!

CHECK IT OUT

Light up now. Take six deep drags and ask yourself what it is that you are actually enjoying.

Isn't it true that it's not so much that you enjoy inhaling obnoxious fumes into your lungs, but that you feel you can't enjoy social occasions, or cope with stress, without them?

BUT DRUGS ARE DIFFICULT TO KICK!

That's only if you believe that you get some genuine pleasure or benefit out of them. Once you realize that not only does smoking damage your health and wealth but it also destroys your nerves and confidence, you can actually enjoy the process of quitting...

IMMEDIATELY AND PERMANENTLY!

WHAT ABOUT THE WITHDRAWAL PANGS?

Although nicotine is the world's most powerful drug going by the speed with which it hooks smokers, you are never badly hooked.

The actual physical withdrawal from nicotine is so slight that smokers only know the feeling as…

I WANT A CIGARETTE!

QUITTING

THOSE CRAVINGS

Nicotine withdrawal is similar to hunger for food. In both cases, you feel irritable and empty when unable to relieve the feeling and you only begin to feel confident, satisfied, and relaxed once you satisfy the hunger or craving.

THE COMPLETE OPPOSITE
OF HUNGER

Good food genuinely tastes good, whereas tobacco tastes foul. Food is survival. Tobacco is death. Food genuinely satisfies hunger, whereas tobacco creates the craving. Eating is a genuine pleasure we can enjoy throughout our lives. Smoking is an illusion of pleasure, an ingenious confidence trick which enslaves us for life.

I ENJOY THE TASTE

Most smokers can remember how foul those first cigarettes tasted and how hard they had to work to inhale. Ask a smoker: "If you can't get your own brand, do you abstain?" A smoker would rather smoke old rope! It's like working on a pig farm. After a while, you become immune to the smell. Smokers become immune to the smell of stale tobacco.

INTRODUCING THE BIG MONSTER

From birth, we are subjected to a massive, daily bombardment telling us that cigarettes relieve boredom and stress, and aid concentration and relaxation. When someone is about to be executed, the last request is always a cigarette. A husband chain-smokes outside the maternity ward. When the baby is born, cigars are handed around in celebration.

THE BRAINWASHING

This is the "big monster" in the mind and the real reason we find it difficult to quit. It doesn't affect us before we are hooked since the beautiful truth is that our lives were complete before we tried those first experimental cigarettes.

But once we do, the "little monster" confirms the brainwashing or, more accurately, fools our brains into believing it.

THE VOID

Our children all seem to be searching for some magical elixir or prop as if the incredible intelligence that created us (be it God or three billion years of natural selection) has omitted some vital ingredient essential to our enjoyment of life, or to our ability to survive.

QUITTIN

THE INCREDIBLE MACHINE

The human body is the most sophisticated survival machine on the planet. It is complete. But children and teenagers have yet to mature. They feel insecure and vulnerable. Little wonder that they turn to illusory props which guarantee they will never mature, unless and until they are free from both monsters.

LIKE CLAUSTROPHOBIA

Try forcing a claustrophobic into a confined space and they will panic. They won't suffocate, but if you believe you will it's the same. If you believe that you can't enjoy life, or handle stress, without a cigarette, you will feel miserable and insecure without one.

QUITTING

THE ITCH

Think of the "little monster" as an almost imperceptible itch that you can partially and temporarily relieve only by lighting up. Like tight shoes, the longer you suffer, the greater the relief. This is why the so-called special cigarettes follow a period of abstinence... after a meal, exercise, sex, or whatever.

THE FIRST OF THE DAY

The one that makes us cough our lungs up, but ironically a favorite for many smokers. It's because we've gone eight hours without nicotine. When we awake we relieve a series of aggravations… our bladders, our thirst, etc. A nonsmoker will relieve his hunger. A smoker is more likely to light a cigarette.

FOOD OR NICOTINE

Although the empty feeling is indistinguishable, nicotine will not relieve hunger for food, or vice versa. This is why I became a chain-smoker. After that first cigarette of the day, I still had the empty feeling which was hunger for food. But to my confused brain it meant: I need another cigarette, and another.

QUITTING

THE TUG OF WAR

All smokers suffer from a permanent tug of war within their minds.

On the one side—

> *It's filthy and disgusting slavery destroying my health and wealth.*

On the other side—

> *It's my friend, my pleasure, my crutch.*

THE REALITY

It's a tug of war of fear. There is no genuine pleasure or crutch. The other side is also fear. The reality is: *How can I enjoy life or cope with life without them?* Both sets of fear are caused by nicotine. Nonsmokers don't suffer from either.

NEITHER WILL YOU ONCE YOU ARE FREE!

I WISH I WAS A HAPPY CASUAL SMOKER

There is no such thing. With a permanent itch, the natural tendency is to scratch it all the time. The natural tendency for smokers is to become a chain-smoker. So why aren't all smokers chain-smokers? Because the effect on our health, wealth, and self-respect makes us try to control our intake of poison.

SMOKE LESS
—HOOKED MORE!

The less you smoke, the less it affects your health and wealth, and the less you desire to quit. The longer you go before scratching the itch, the greater the illusion of pleasure, or crutch, and the greater your desire to continue smoking.

I CAN GO A WEEK WITHOUT SMOKING

If there is genuine pleasure, why would you want to? If there is none, why smoke at all?

I can go for a week without carrots, but feel no need to boast about it. Perhaps I would boast if I'd had to discipline myself and deprive myself for a whole week. If we are proud of how little we smoke, just think how great it will feel to be free!

ALL SMOKERS LIE TO THEMSELVES

Why? Because we sense that we've fallen into a trap and feel stupid and weak-willed because we've failed to escape from it. So we give phoney reasons to justify our stupidity in order to retain some semblance of self-respect. No way do we deceive nonsmokers. We don't even deceive ourselves.

I ONLY ENJOY TWO A DAY

So why do you smoke the others?

In fact you never enjoy any.

This is why the vast majority of cigarettes are smoked subconsciously. If every time you lit a cigarette, you had to be aware of the $130,000/£100,000 you spend, the filth in your lungs, and that this might just be the one to trigger off lung cancer, even the illusion of enjoyment would go.

WHY DO SMOKERS
FIND IT HARD TO QUIT?

It's because the two monsters have fooled them into believing that they are making a genuine sacrifice, that a meal will never be as enjoyable, that they won't be able to handle stress, that they have to go through a transitional period of misery, and that, even if they succeed, they will have to resist temptation for the rest of their lives.

QUITTING

THE EFFECTS OF
BRAINWASHING

Think of the umpteen smokers who quit for ten years then started again or are still moping about how they miss cigarettes. Or ex-smokers who tell you how great they feel and who next time you see them are puffing away again. Think of smokers who are clearly killing themselves yet still smoke, as well as the misery of your own failed attempts when using willpower.

THE WILLPOWER METHOD

Something triggers off an attempt to quit. The smoker embarks on a period of abstinence, like a child being deprived of its sweets, hoping that, if he has the willpower to resist the temptation long enough, one day he will wake up with the feeling:

"EUREKA! I'M FREE!!!"

QUITTING

WHY HE NEVER ACHIEVES IT

After a few days the congestion goes, you have more money, no longer despise yourself, and have that wonderful holier-than-thou feeling of no longer being a slave. All the reasons that made you decide to quit are rapidly disappearing. Meanwhile, the "little monster" hasn't had his fix—your brain is saying:

"I WANT A CIGARETTE!"

THE CONFUSION

For some mysterious reason, you still want a cigarette but aren't allowed to have one. You start to feel deprived and miserable. This is one of the occasions when your brain has been programmed to light up a cigarette, so you feel even more miserable. Soon your whole life is dominated by the misery of not being allowed to smoke.

EVENTUALLY YOUR WILLPOWER RUNS OUT

You get fed up with always feeling miserable. You start searching for reasons to have just one cigarette and eventually you find one. The longer you've abstained, the weirder the taste of that first cigarette. The longer you have suffered the misery of feeling deprived, the greater the illusion of pleasure. You are soon back where you started.

QUITTING

ABSENCE MAKES THE HEART GROW FONDER

If you believe there is some genuine pleasure in smoking, why should that belief ever disappear? The "little monster" works just like normal hunger and normal stress. This means that long after the "little monster" has died, during times of normal hunger or stress the ex-smoker's brain is still fooled into believing that a cigarette will help.

IT'S CONFLICT NOT LACK OF WILLPOWER

At our clinics we ask smokers who think they are weak-willed: *If you ran out late at night, how far would you walk for a packet of cigarettes?*

A smoker would swim across the Mississippi river for a packet. A strong-willed child will keep its tantrum going forever. It takes a strong-willed person to block their mind to the terrible health risks involved and continue to smoke.

I KNEW THAT I
WAS STRONG-WILLED

I couldn't understand why no one and nothing else in my life controlled me, yet I was completely dominated by something I loathed, or why my friends could smoke ten a day and I had to chain-smoke. It never occurred to me that they couldn't afford to chain-smoke, or that their lungs couldn't cope with the poison.

NATIONAL NO SMOKING DAY

According to the media, this is the day every smoker attempts to quit. But in reality this is the day every smoker smokes twice as many and twice as blatantly as before because smokers don't like being told what to do by people who don't understand. It takes a strong-willed person to resist the massive pressures that smokers are subjected to today.

QUITTING

CHECK OUT YOUR SMOKING FRIENDS

You'll find that your acquaintances who are still heavy smokers are strong-willed. But we are about to remove any conflict of wills.

HOW DOES "EASYWAY" WORK?

By simply removing the confusion and misconceptions that make it difficult to quit. Smokers try to "give up" smoking. This implies a genuine sacrifice. For the reasons I have already explained, there is absolutely nothing to give up.

The two monsters create the illusion of providing pleasure or a crutch. The reality is the complete opposite.

QUITTIN

THE ADVANTAGES
OF BEING A SMOKER

There aren't any. I don't mean the disadvantages outweigh them. I mean there is no pleasure or crutch whatsoever. On the contrary, smoking destroys your nerves and confidence, and creates boredom, restlessness, and dissatisfaction. Far from being your friend, it would be difficult to imagine a worse enemy.

IT'S FEAR THAT KEEPS US SMOKING

One subtlety of the nicotine trap is that it keeps its victims trapped for life.

You might feel that I'm taking away and giving nothing back. You might be tempted to stop reading or to abandon your attempt. Please don't fall for the trap. Like me, the majority of ex-smokers that used my method found it to be the most rewarding experience of their lives.

SNUFF-TAKING

Sniffing dried tobacco is a form of nicotine addiction. Like smoking, it was regarded as a habit. Addicts used similar gimmicks to disguise the filth like silver snuff-boxes. Do heroin addicts enjoy injections? Do cocaine-sniffers enjoy sniffing for sniffing's sake, or are these just the rather disgusting methods we use to administer the drug?

I ENJOY THE RITUAL

Smokers believe that there is an actual pleasure in smoking and that the health risks and expense are merely hazards that interfere with that pleasure. If that were true, smokers would enjoy herbal cigarettes. They never do. Smoking is merely a more dangerous and disgusting form of nicotine addiction.

A MOMENT TO REFLECT

If you are not yet convinced that there is nothing to give up and that the pleasure, or crutch, from smoking is merely an ingenious confidence trick, it is essential that you stop reading at this stage, go back to the beginning, and start again. Remember, I have nothing but good news for you, provided you follow my instructions.

QUITTING

WHAT ARE YOU TRYING TO ACHIEVE?

Never to smoke again? No. This is what smokers who use willpower do. They go through the rest of their lives hoping they'll never smoke again. Which means they don't achieve their object until they die. This means they never know whether or not they succeeded.

WHEN DO YOU BECOME
A NONSMOKER?

It is important that you reflect on this question.
Typical answers are:

> When I stop thinking about smoking.
> *How do you stop thinking about it?*

> When I can enjoy a meal or answer the
> phone etc. without craving a cigarette.
> *How long will that be?*

> When I've quit for a year.
> *Why wait a year? Why not longer?*

It's all so vague and indecisive.

WHAT YOU ARE TRYING TO ACHIEVE!

The real difference between a smoker and a nonsmoker is not that the latter doesn't smoke but that he or she has no desire to smoke. If you have no desire to smoke, there is no temptation to smoke, and therefore no need for willpower to resist the temptation.

A FRAME OF MIND

What you are trying to achieve is a frame of mind, so that when you extinguish the final cigarette, for the next few days, and for the rest of your life, whenever you think about smoking, instead of thinking: "I'd love a cigarette," or "When will I be free?", you say to yourself:

"EUREKA! I'M ALREADY FREE!

I'M A NONSMOKER!"

HOW WILL YOU KNOW THAT YOU ARE FREE?

By clearing up all the doubts and confusion before you extinguish the final cigarette. By realizing that there is no such thing as special or occasional cigarettes but a lifetime's chain of misery. By realizing that you are giving up nothing. On the contrary, you are receiving marvelous, positive gains.

QUITTI

THOSE MARVELOUS, POSITIVE GAINS

I knew I was almost literally burning my hard-earned money and risking terrible diseases. The chain reaction was like a time bomb ticking away inside my body. I never knew the length of the fuse; I just hoped I would quit before it went off. It's great to be free of the fear and self-despising, but there were even greater unexpected gains.

THE LETHARGY

I knew the coughing and congestion were due to smoking, but I thought the lack of energy was down to old age. I struggled to get up in the morning and fell asleep each evening watching TV. It's great to wake up full of energy after having a good night's rest, actually wanting to exercise, and feeling young again.

THE FEAR

As a youth I enjoyed medicals, believing I was indestructible. As a smoker I hated them. I even hated visiting other people in hospitals. The mere thought of chest X-rays would create panic. I was convinced that cigarettes gave me courage. It's so great to feel strong again, to be able to enjoy the good times, and to feel fully equipped to cope with the bad.

QUITTING

THE SLAVERY

So intent was I on resisting all the attempts of the do-gooders who were trying to inform me of what I already knew—**SMOKERS ARE FOOLS!**—it never occurred to me that I spent half my life feeling miserable because I wasn't allowed to smoke, and the other half being miserable because I did.

IT'S SO LOVELY BEING FREE!

QUITTING

IS SMOKING A SOCIABLE PASTIME?

In the old days you could visit a strange office or a friend's house and ask: "Do you mind if I smoke?" It was really a polite way of asking for an ashtray. Ask for an ashtray now and people look at you as if you're requesting some relic from the distant past. Smokers regard themselves as social pariahs.

THE SINISTER BLACK SHADOW

All our lives the fear of quitting makes us block our minds to the bad effects of smoking. It's like an ever-increasing black shadow forming in our sub-conscious. Strong people loathe being controlled by something they hate. The greatest gain is to be free of this dark cloud and the self-loathing that goes with it, and to genuinely pity rather than envy smokers.

UITTING

THE FIRST POWERFUL INFLUENCE

Before I started smoking, life was exciting. I could enjoy the highs and handle the stresses. When I finally discovered the "EASYWAY" to quit, it was like waking from a nightmare, escaping from a black-and-white world of fear and depression into a sunshine world of health, confidence, and freedom. I still can't get over the euphoria.

THE SECOND POWERFUL INFLUENCE

All creatures on this planet instinctively know the difference between food and poison. Even before that first experimental cigarette, we know that there is something evil and unnatural about breathing lethal fumes into our lungs. To have to do it all day every day because of the influence of a subtle, sinister drug is not only evil but ought to be unthinkable.

THE CORRECT DECISION

Some decisions are difficult to make. How can you be certain that a particular car or TV is the best value for you? However, there is one decision in your life which is easy to make: whether to spend the rest of your life as a smoker or a nonsmoker. Smoking provides no advantages whatsoever and horrendous disadvantages.

IF YOU HESITATE

It's not because you are too stupid to see the obvious, you don't even need me to tell you the correct decision, it is because of **FEAR!** The greatest gain is to be free of that fear—it's caused by the drug. You never decided to become a smoker, but fell into an ingenious trap that is designed to enslave you for life.

THE INGENUITY OF THE TRAP

We are fooled into believing we smoke because it offers genuine pleasure or a crutch. Therefore we don't decide to quit until we have genuine stress in our lives, like a shortage of money or bad health. But these are exactly the times we most need our little *"friend."* If we quit, the reasons for doing so soon disappear, so we start smoking again.

WHY THE TIME
WILL NEVER BE RIGHT

Because the times you most need to quit are the times you most need your little *"friend."* Because there will always be some occasion shortly coming up in your life, be it social or work-related, to enable you to put off the evil day. That is part of the ingenuity of the trap. Be aware of it! Don't fall for it!

QUITTIN

SOME SMOKERS
JUST DRIFT OUT OF IT

Rather like they drifted into it. I waited 33 years hoping that
would happen to me. Believe me, it will no more happen
than you are likely to drift out of a bear trap. You will only
escape if you make a positive effort to do so, and the first
step is to take the decision to make that attempt. I want
you to do that now.

IT TAKES COURAGE

I want you to have the courage to make that decision now. I'm not asking you to smoke your final cigarette now—I'll advise you when to do that—but merely to make the decision that you'll go for it. If you have the courage to do that, and follow my instructions to the letter, you will not only find it easy but enjoyable.

A FEELING OF DOOM AND GLOOM

If you have one, dismiss it now. You are about to achieve something marvelous, something that every smoker on the planet would love to achieve: **TO BE FREE!** You are on a winner to nothing. If you don't succeed, you are no worse off. But let's not even think about failure. Start right now with a feeling of excitement, challenge, and elation.

HOW DO I COPE WITH THE WITHDRAWAL?

The actual physical withdrawal from nicotine is no worse when you quit than the pangs you suffer throughout your regular smoking life. Although nicotine is the world's most powerful drug to judge by the speed with which it hooks you, fortunately you are never badly hooked. The physical discomfort disappears after about five days. After three weeks, you cease to be addicted.

QUITTING

SO WHY DO SMOKERS GET SO IRRITABLE?

It's for exactly the same reason they get into a panic when they run out of cigarettes. Smokers don't wake up in a panic even though they've gone eight hours without nicotine. Most smokers nowadays will leave the bedroom or eat breakfast before they light their first cigarette. Others will wait until they arrive at work.

THAT FEELING OF PANIC

It can start even before you run out. You're at a party and ration out your cigarettes, saving one to go to bed with and one for the morning. Some joker says: "Do you mind if I have one?" As you meekly hand it over you're thinking: "Mind? Of course I mind! I'll gladly give you a pint of blood, I might even donate a kidney, but not my last cigarette!"

ADDICTION IS MENTAL NOT PHYSICAL

The almost imperceptible physical discomfort created by the "little monster" acts as a catalyst which triggers off the "big monster." It is the "big monster" which creates the fear and panic—the belief that we cannot enjoy or cope with life without nicotine. Fortunately, we can remove the illusion, fear, and panic prior to the final cigarette.

BE AWARE OF THE "LITTLE MONSTER"

For a few days after quitting, the "little monster" will live on. You might be aware of a feeling of insecurity, or merely: "I want a cigarette." This is when ex-smokers get confused and miserable because they can't have one. They believe they are being deprived of a genuine pleasure or crutch.

BE PREPARED FOR THAT FEELING

But don't worry about it. Recognize it for what it is. Say to yourself: *"It's what smokers feel throughout their smoking lives and what keeps them miserable, poor, lethargic, unhealthy slaves!"*

Rejoice in the fact that you have already escaped from the prison. Revel in the death throes of the "little monster!"

ESCAPED OR
TRYING TO ESCAPE?

You become a nonsmoker
the moment you extinguish your
final cigarette. *But how do you
know it is your final cigarette?* The
answer is, simply by removing all doubts and uncertainty first. If
you have doubts, you are hoping not to smoke again. How will you
ever know? You'll be waiting for nothing to happen and, like so
many ex-smokers, will do so the rest of your life.

QUITTIN

BUT HOW CAN YOU EVER
BE CERTAIN?

Would you take up a pastime which gave you no pleasure or advantages whatsoever, that cost you a fortune, shortened your life, and made you feel nervous, lethargic, unclean, stupid, and miserable? The biggest idiot on earth wouldn't! Having made what you know to be the correct decision, never punish yourself by ever doubting it!

OH, I'D LOVE A CIGARETTE!

How often do you hear ex-smokers, whether they have quit for a few hours, days, or even years, make similar statements? It is these whining stoppers that make existing smokers frightened even to make the attempt—they share the harmful belief of once a smoker always a smoker, that once addicted you can never be completely free!

IT'S ABSOLUTE NONSENSE!!!

HOW STUPID CAN YOU GET?

Why does an otherwise intelligent person decide to quit, then spend the rest of their life bemoaning the fact that they can't smoke the occasional cigarette? It's because they doubt their decision; they believe they have made a genuine sacrifice, and that they gained some genuine pleasure or crutch from smoking.

IN REALITY
IT'S EVEN MORE STUPID!

What they are moping for never actually existed. For example, the favorite cigarette, like the one after a meal. Can you ever actually remember thinking: *"This really tastes marvelous!"?*

Isn't it true that it's not so much that we enjoy smoking, but more that we assume we do because we are miserable without cigarettes?

REMEMBER THOSE STRESSFUL SITUATIONS

When your car broke down in the pouring rain in the middle of nowhere and, soaking wet and covered in grease, can you remember lighting up and thinking: *"I'm late for the most important appointment of my life. But who cares. I've got this gorgeous packet of cigarettes!"*

Did they make you genuinely happy?

I CAN'T ANSWER THE PHONE WITHOUT ONE

This is a common plea of the many powerful business executives who attend our clinics. What's so stressful about the phone? It won't blow up, or bite you. It's that little itch that's causing the stress. That's also why smokers find it difficult to concentrate without first removing the distraction. Nonsmokers don't suffer from the problem.

BUT IT DEFINITELY RELIEVES BOREDOM

Does it? Boredom is a frame of mind. When you smoke a cigarette do you sit there thinking: "Oh, how mind-absorbing and fascinating this is?" Can you think of anything more boring than chain-smoking cigarette after cigarette, day in day out, for 33 years as I once did? We smoke when bored because there is nothing to distract us from the itch.

NEVER DOUBT YOUR DECISION

It's the uncertainty that makes it difficult to quit. Having made what you know to be the correct decision, never punish yourself by questioning that decision. If you see one cigarette as a pleasure or crutch, you'll see a million cigarettes that way. By craving one, you'll be miserable because you can't have it and you'll be even more miserable if you do!

THE GREATEST MISTAKE

When they try to quit, many smokers attempt not to think about smoking. This merely creates a phobia. Remember, something marvelous is happening. It's what you are thinking that's important. If it's: "I can't have one," or "When will I be free?," you'll be doubting your decision. Instead always think:

"YIPPEE! I'M A NONSMOKER!!!"

"THE MOMENT OF REVELATION"

If you follow the instructions, after just a few days you'll have a moment—it might be a social or stressful situation, one of those times that you thought you could never enjoy or handle without a cigarette—when not only did you enjoy or handle it, but you never even thought about smoking. That's when you know you are free!

DON'T WAIT FOR IT TO HAPPEN

If you try to force "The Moment of Revelation," it will be like worrying about not being able to sleep, you'll merely ensure it won't happen. You become a nonsmoker the moment you cut off the supply of nicotine. Just get on with your life. Accept that you'll have good days and bad just as smokers do.

DON'T CHANGE YOUR LIFESTYLE

Don't avoid smoking friends just because you've quit smoking. If you do, you'll be miserable. Remember, you aren't giving up living. You aren't giving up anything. On the contrary, as your energy level and confidence soar, you'll find your capacity to enjoy life and to handle stress will improve.

IT ALL HAPPENS SO SLOWLY

Another ingenuity of the nicotine trap is that our slide down the pit is so gradual we aren't even aware of the increasing decline in our physical and mental health. The problem is that, when we quit, recovery is gradual and, if we are using the willpower method and thus are feeling deprived, we tend not to see the immense gains.

IT TAKES SEVEN YEARS TO CLEAR THE CONTAMINATION FROM YOUR BODY

Or every cigarette you smoke takes five minutes off your life. Both the above statements are true but only if you contract one of the killer diseases. If you quit now, your health will recover to 99% of what it would have been if you'd never been a smoker, and the bulk of the contamination leaves in the first few days and weeks.

USE YOUR IMAGINATION

If it were possible to project any smoker three weeks into the future to give them a sense of how they will feel without cigarettes, not just physically but confidence-wise, they would have no hesitation in quitting cheerfully and immediately. I can't do that, but you can!

JUST USE YOUR IMAGINATION!

TIME IS ON YOUR SIDE

Providing you've removed the brainwashing first, once you've cut off the supply of nicotine, nothing can prevent you from being free. You will already be a nonsmoker and it is essential that you think of yourself as one immediately. Otherwise, you could find yourself waiting forever.

EXPECT SOME DISORIENTATION

Even changes for the better, like a new job, house or car, involve a period of adjustment. If you do feel strange at first, that will soon go provided you don't start worrying about it. Remember, any slight aggravation you might suffer is not because you've quit but because you started in the first place. Nonsmokers don't suffer from withdrawal.

I KEEP FORGETTING I'VE QUIT

Don't worry! It's quite normal and a good sign. It means that already your mind isn't completely obsessed with smoking. But these are the times when willpower stoppers start to doubt and mope. Train yourself to send doubts packing immediately; remind yourself how lucky you are to be free, or just say: "YIPPEE, I'M A NONSMOKER!" That way, those moments become pleasure.

I CAN'T GET UP WITHOUT A CIGARETTE

When you extinguish that final cigarette, look forward to being free for the rest of the day. Lie in bed reflecting that you have already achieved the most difficult part—you have made a start and are now able to anticipate the exciting challenge of proving you can not only survive but actually enjoy a whole day, from dawn to dusk, **FREE!!!**

IT HAPPENS ON SOCIAL OCCASIONS

You're chatting away oblivious. Then the cigarettes are handed round. You find yourself subconsciously taking one. Your friend smirks: "I thought you'd given up!" You feel stupid. Don't just stand there. Instead say: "I'd quite forgotten." (Which is all that happened.) "I can't tell you how lovely it is to be free. You should try it!" Hand the cigarette back. The situation is now reversed.

YOU HOLD THE ACES

There is a constant battle between smokers and ex-smokers. As more and more smokers leave the sinking ship, those left behind feel more stupid, insecure, and isolated. This fear can cause even people that love you to try to get you hooked again. Never forget that the ex-smoker holds all the aces and the smoker doesn't even have a pair of twos!

ATTEND SOCIAL FUNCTIONS IMMEDIATELY

Even if you are the only nonsmoker present (usually the reverse nowadays), always be aware that every one of those smokers would love to be like you. They will expect you to be miserable. When they see you happy and cheerful, they'll think you are Superman or Superwoman.

The important point is…
YOU'LL FEEL A MILLION DOLLARS!
ENJOY YOUR ESCAPE!

WHEN WILL THE CRAVING GO?

The "little monster" causes the physical itch to your body. But it is only your brain that is capable of craving a cigarette. For a few days the "little monster" might continue to trigger the thought: "I want a cigarette." Your brain has the choice of craving one, or instead recognizing the feeling for what it is and saying: **"YIPPEE! I'M A NONSMOKER!!!"**

WHEN A FRIEND OR RELATIVE DIES

You have to go through a period of mourning. Eventually time partially heals the wound and life goes on. It's the same with the willpower stoppers. If they can suffer the misery long enough, life goes on. But they still believe they've given up a genuine pleasure or crutch. Come a trauma in their lives, smoke one cigarette—they're back in the trap!

QUITTIN

WHEN AN ENEMY DIES

You don't have to go through a mourning process. You can rejoice immediately and for the rest of your life. The cigarette was never a friend. It was the worst disease you'll ever suffer from. You have it under control. Now you have the choice of spending the next few days moping over an illusion or rejoicing:

"YIPPEE! I'M A NONSMOKER!!!"

I NEED A SUBSTITUTE

I presume that you are searching for some elixir that will have contradictory effects like relieving boredom and helping concentration, relieving stress, and improving relaxation, which at the same time won't destroy your health and wealth. If you ever find it, please let me know. By the way, why don't you search for Aladdin's lamp while you're at it?

DO NOT USE SUBSTITUTES

By even searching for something to take the place of smoking you confirm that you are making a sacrifice—*there is a void in my life. I need something to take its place.* When you get rid of a bout of influenza, do you search for a substitute disease? Nicotine created the void. You didn't need to smoke before you became hooked. Substitutes merely prolong the feeling of a void.

WILL I PUT ON WEIGHT?

You only gain weight if you substitute sweets or gum for smoking or start picking between meals. Not only will you get fat and miserable, but you won't even satisfy the empty feeling and will prolong your search for illusory rewards. If you put on a couple of pounds due to having a better appetite, don't worry. When you've kicked smoking, you can beat anything.

WILL NICOTINE GUM OR PATCHES HELP?

NO! In theory while you are breaking the habit they ease the terrible physical withdrawal pains and when you've broken the habit you wean yourself off the nicotine substitute. In fact the physical withdrawal is almost imperceptible and it's not habit but addiction. They keep the "little monster" alive and keep the "big monster" craving!

QUITTING

ENJOY HAVING A NONSMOKE

If you cannot visualize certain activities without smoking, break the association from the start. Have your drink, do your crossword, whatever. Enjoy not smoking. Enjoy not only removing the contamination from your body, but also proving that you can easily enjoy life without smoking. It's only smokers who can't enjoy life without nicotine.

I'LL HAVE TO GIVE UP GOLF

I couldn't visualize ever wanting to play without smoking. In fact I couldn't visualize life without cigarettes. Now I can't visualize that I was once a nicotine slave. Soon you'll find it difficult to understand why you ever felt the need to smoke, and wonder why you can't make other smokers appreciate just how nice it is to be free!

OBSERVE CASUAL SMOKERS AT PARTIES

They almost chain-smoke! Notice how agitated they are when not smoking. Watch the obvious relief when they light up. Observe how quickly the cigarette burns and watch the increasing agitation when the nicotine wears off. Remember that tomorrow they have to continue the chain ad infinitum for life!

OBSERVE SMOKERS GENERALLY

Watch teenagers smoking in the street, drivers in a heavy traffic jam, office workers outside a nonsmoking office, holiday-makers whose flight has been delayed, or lone smokers at a social function. Notice they don't even seem to be aware that they are smoking, how much more miserable they look, and how even much more miserable they are when not allowed to smoke.

TIMING

When you quit, the natural tendency is to pick a period when you feel you least need a cigarette. Like practically every other aspect of smoking, the correct course to take is the complete opposite of what you'd expect. Start at a time you consider to be the most difficult, prove immediately that you can enjoy the social occasion, or handle the stress, and the rest is easy.

ITTING

A DEGENERATING DISEASE

With a disease that gets worse and worse, it doesn't take Sherlock Holmes to deduce that the quicker you get rid of it, the better. If you had Alzheimer's or Parkinson's disease and there were a simple cure, would you delay a single day? Smoking is the No.1 killer disease in society, but fortunately there is a simple cure…

STOP NOW!

THE FINAL PREPARATION

You should now be like a dog straining at the leash to smoke that final cigarette. If not, there can only be two reasons: that you do not believe that smoking confers no advantages whatsoever—if so, read back from the beginning—or that you believe this, but still have a feeling of doom and gloom. In which case, stop being dumb and trust me.

THE FINAL CIGARETTE

I want you to smoke your final cigarette, not with a feeling of doom and gloom, but with a feeling of elation. Did you decide to fall into the trap? Just think how great the Count of Monte Cristo felt when he finally escaped from that prison. Don't extinguish that final cigarette thinking: "I must never smoke again." Rather…

"ISN'T IT MARVELOUS? I DON'T EVER NEED TO EVER AGAIN!"

NEVER ENVY SMOKERS

You are not being deprived. If you see someone smoking, no matter what the occasion, be aware that they are not smoking because they choose to. They are being deprived of their money, health, energy, relaxation, self-respect, and freedom. All that, to achieve what? Nothing! Just trying to feel like a nonsmoker. Smokers are drug addicts and, like all drug addiction, it'll just get worse and worse.

HELP THEM! PITY THEM!

TELL ALLEN CARR'S EASYWAY ORGANIZATION
THAT YOU'VE ESCAPED

Leave a comment on www.allencarr.com,
like our Facebook page www.facebook.com/AllenCarr or write to
the Worldwide Head Office at the address shown below.

....

ALLEN CARR'S EASYWAY CENTERS

The success rate at the centers, based on the three-month, money-back guarantee, is over 90 percent. Selected centers also offer sessions that deal with alcohol, other drugs, and weight issues. Please check with your nearest center for details. Allen Carr's Easyway guarantees that you will find it easy to stop at the centers or your money back.

ALLEN CARR'S EASYWAY
Worldwide Head Office

Park House, 14 Pepys Road,
Raynes Park, London
SW20 8NH ENGLAND
Tel: +44 (0)208 9447761
Email: mail@allencarr.com
Website: www.allencarr.com

Worldwide Press Office

Tel: +44 (0)7970 88 44 52
Email: media@allencarr.com

Allen Carr's Easway method has helped tens of millions of people to quit smoking, alcohol, illicit drugs, gambling, and overspending, as well as to deal with sugar addiction, overeating, and fear of flying. For further information, including details of Allen Carr centers worldwide as well as live/online seminars and issues the method addresses, please visit allencarr.com